FINDING M.E.

KATIE MANNING

Copyright © 2015 Katie Manning

All rights reserved.

ISBN-13: 978-1516935956

ISBN-10: 1516935950

To Australia- for helping me come out of my shell.

To my astounding CFS community- for being you and for showing me the meaning of strength.

CONTENTS

	Gratitude	i
1	Prologue	1
2	What The Hell Is Going On?	7
3	Is This Really Happening?	26
4	Moving On Up	39
5	Taking A Tumble	47
6	A Change Of Scenery	56
7	An Ongoing Experience	73
8	Closing	82
9	Resources	84
	About The Author	85

GRATITUDE

Thank you first and foremost to CFS for teaching me so many valuable lessons and for really enabling me to stretch myself in ways I never thought possible.

Thank you to my beautiful friends, Tara Bliss and Ali Coleman, for keeping me going with my writing and always believing in me.

Thank you to all of my gorgeous volunteer proof-readers- I couldn't have done it without you.

Thank you to the MacDonald clan for making me feel at home.

Thank you so much Mum, Dad, James and the Manning tribe- I can't really find the words to express how grateful I am. I got there in the end, didn't I?!

Fraz, my man- you're such a legend. Thank you for being my husband, my partner-in-crime, my own personal stand-up comic and for continuing to give me amazing advice, even when I'm too stubborn to hear it. I'm learning though…!

CHAPTER 1
PROLOGUE

It wasn't supposed to be like this, not in your twenties. Living in the body of a 95-year-old woman when I should've been downing melon-flavoured shots with anonymous faces at 3 o'clock in the morning.

All week, I'd denied that anything was happening, putting it down to a bad dose of flu, but when I woke up feeling like my bones had been shattered one-by-one in an imaginary car accident, even I, the famously stubborn one, had to admit that something was a little off. I didn't want to move a muscle for fear that I would smash into a million pieces, for fear that my body would melt away. I was utterly, *utterly* exhausted. My throat was tired, my feet were tired, even my eyelashes and eyebrows felt tired. I couldn't even admit there might be a *slight* problem when my only way of getting to the bathroom solo was crawling on my stomach and having to stop for breaks on the 2-metre journey from my University hall bed to the bathroom. My whole body had ground to a halt with a sudden, nauseating jolt as if I was the only one who didn't see the stop sign, as if somehow everyone knew that this would happen eventually. I couldn't ask for help though- how would I even begin to ask for help if I genuinely thought I was going insane?

This was just the very, very beginning of my journey with M.E. (Myalgic Encephalomyelitis), an illness which often goes by the name of CFS (Chronic Fatigue Syndrome). Whether you believe that M.E. and CFS are different or separate illnesses, labels don't seem to really help us when we're stuck in the thick of it. Fatigue in all of its forms is a symptom of our times- a society in which we fill our lives with 'busy' to make us feel adequate and to show people we are successful and admirable; in which we constantly convince ourselves that we're ok just to stifle our true selves that little bit further and make sure we don't upset anyone; a life in which caring for yourself seems to be synonymous with pure, unadulterated selfishness and narrow-mindedness.

Before having spent most of my twenties (and a few years before that) wiped out by this debilitating illness, I had absolutely no idea about how little I respected and thought of myself. I had no idea just how many people are unknowingly affected by fatigue on a daily basis, and how their reaction to this imbalance is often a reflection of their attitude towards life and self-love. In reading and hearing people's reactions to M.E./CFS as a 'made up' illness and an illness that is only in the mind, not the body, I've had to ride through the whole spectrum of emotions- total apathy, rage, anger, disappointment, acknowledgement, acceptance, understanding and love.

I think the cloud lifted when I gradually began to piece my life together again by restarting University and trying to maintain my energy levels, but I'm making this sound a lot easier than it actually was. Relapses became increasingly difficult to take. I didn't learn any of the lessons they had to teach me until much later in my recovery journey and I often wondered if I would fall into the same mental state that I was in before.

Now, I'm pleased and grateful to say that I have a better outlook that I had even before I was sick. This doesn't mean that it's always smooth-sailing and I'm not walking around in a bubble thinking I'm oblivious to life's difficulties. I just believe that having lived through CFS, I now have a better emotional toolkit to be able to deal with these little niggles. My hope is that you can become equipped with your *own* emotional toolkit as well.

In short, I've learned more about myself and others through having this illness than I think I'll ever learn in this lifetime. If you asked me whether I'd go back and change anything, I wouldn't swap this experience for the world. The reason people use this cliché after serious illness is because the best clichés are often true. I haven't always looked on sickness so favourably, but as Steve Jobs so pointedly observed, "You can't connect the dots looking forward; you can only connect them looking backwards. So you have to trust that the dots will somehow connect in your future."

Even though you might have heard this quote dozens of time, I still feel a lump in my throat whenever I read or hear it. This elegantly expressed sentiment sits at the foundation of my learning from my time with M.E./CFS. After being free of the illness and in the best health of my life for the last 5 years, I know that my history of being ill with tiredness and overwhelm is long gone. I'm often asked how I know this for sure, and it's all about connecting those intuitive dots and signposts.

Can you *really* recover from Chronic Fatigue Syndrome?

I have to really put my neck on the line here and say 'yes'- it is possible to fully recovery from Chronic Fatigue Syndrome. I know that some of you might disagree with me, and I understand your point of view. I have read and spoken to countless others who went through exactly the same thing as me, and you'd be absolutely amazed at what they're managing to achieve in life. Like me, they have more energy now than they've ever had before in their lives. They're not going to tell you that it was an easy road, but they are embracing life like never before.

If you'd asked me when I was right in the thick of it all if I thought there was a way out, I definitely would've said 'no'- how can you even *begin* to imagine that symptoms that are so persistent, difficult and misunderstood aren't going to follow you around for the rest of your life? A lot of people believe that because there's no cure for CFS/M.E. (yet), you shouldn't tell people that you're recovered or healed, but I feel it with every part of my body that my illness is not coming back. Every illness and experience is deeply personal, but if anything about the introduction to my book has sparked something in you, I encourage you to keep on reading and take it all in with an open mind and heart. You might just uncover something unexpected.

What to expect from this book

This book is made up of three sections: the first part tells you all about the onset of my symptoms and my diagnosis; the second part is all about how I tried to get better and how I coped with relapses, and the final part is about what happened when I moved from the U.K. to Australia, the final parts of my healing and what life looks like now.

My wish with this book is not to preach to you. This is not a how-to manual and there are no quick-fix solutions. If easy, 'get-well-quick' tricks interest you, then maybe there's another book out there for you with your name all over it. I'm interested in helping you to understand how you might be able to, like me, carve out your own healing journey in which I didn't undertake any traditional medical treatments, but tripped myself up and fell over more times than I care to admit. If you're fed up of searching and interested in creating a lasting, healthy future, then I hope you'll find the key to your own wellness in the pages of this book. What worked for me might not work for you and you might heal a little more quickly than I did, but let this book be the cornerstone to some fascinating insights.

I cannot promise that this book will heal you- I have no professional medical training. We'll have a lot more inner work to do before we get 'there'. But I *can* promise you that there is a light at the end of that tunnel you feel as though you collapsed in a long time ago. I felt wretched, hopeless and completely lost too, until I realised that I was the one holding all the cards.

Let me pull up a chair next to you, hand you a gorgeous, chintzy cup of tea and take you through it.

CHAPTER 2
WHAT THE HELL IS GOING ON?

I would love to be able to tell you that my childhood was one in which I instinctively knew that there was more going on in this life than meets the eye, that I was psychic or that I saw visions of angels and spirits, but that wasn't me. My childhood however *was* one of adventure- family trips to castles at weekends around the North-East of England, sing-alongs in the car, concerts and hot scones, all those little things that you never seem to be able to appreciate as they're happening, but come to feel so grateful for later on in life. I think it's known as a 'foundation'.

From a very early age, I seemed to get the impression from my teachers that I was a little slow in many academic areas. It was only when we moved house at age 9, that I discovered I wasn't as far behind as it appeared at the time, much to the relief of my parents. I soon discovered that I really loved to study and became incredibly curious about everything. My Grandad collected fossils and gemstones for me, I started ballet and piano lessons, wrote for the school newspaper and started handwriting a book decorated in huge, yellow stars about a girl whose magical saxophone granted her wishes every time she played it (it would have been on the New York Times Bestseller list if I'd finished it, trust me on this one!). I soon discovered that I actually wasn't too bad at studying and regularly shut myself in my room to finish off a Geography project or read when I probably should've been spending a little more time messing around outside or playing.

This introversion (by no means a bad thing, by the way) continued into high school, where I retreated even further into my cave as a way of coping with meeting new people. From a familiar, cosy bubble of friends at a village primary school to being spat out to mingle and mix with a thousand other confident faces, study and reading became ways to conserve my energy and deal with those in my class who seemed to like to point out to everyone else that I was a little different. At the time, I didn't really see it as bullying and just buried myself away and kept busy. This name-calling nevertheless followed me and it was only after joining our school choir that I suddenly started to notice I might be being bullied.

Having later trained as high school teacher, I can now look

back on this whole experience and say that I should have spoken up sooner. I used to deliberately get things wrong in my homework, so that the person next to me wouldn't tease me for being a 'swot'. However, the ball always inevitably swung in the other direction when my classmate now alerted everyone to the fact that I was a loser. I couldn't win. It all came to a head one night when my highly intuitive Mum made me admit that something was up. I remember sliding down the radiator in the kitchen, imaging what my friends and classmates would say if word got out that I'd bragged. Would they disown me? How would I cope with it? Would they sit next to me on the bus tomorrow?

I truly believe that my studies saved me, not only from beating myself up about the situation I found myself in at school, but also to cementing what I had known for a while, that Languages and Music, words and harmonies, were my thing.

The last two years of high school were where I really came into my own. I suddenly rediscovered a group of friends I'd 'lost' a few years earlier and was the first person to bring tank tops back on the Sixth Form style scene (indeed). I studied English Literature, French, German and Music and was incredibly happy. Even though I'd chosen very wordy, 'in your head' subjects, they were balanced out by Music, the subject I was destined to study at University.

Ever since I'd started singing in the school choir, something inside me had changed. I suddenly became more self-accepting and wasn't afraid to sing out. I could hide my voice and blend in with everyone around me for the first time in my life. Even though I had come from a long line of singers and musicians, I think my family and I presumed that this talent had skipped a generation, so always thought of choir as just a bit of socialising and a chance to have fun.

It came as quite a shock then when within two years, I had given up dancing lessons and become one of the youngest members of our local County Choir. I was then invited to sing with numerous University choirs whilst still in high school, before auditioning and becoming a member of the National Youth Choir. I toured, sang for BBC television and radio, and found myself in the Albert Hall dressing rooms quite regularly. The stage was set, so to speak.

It turned out though that choosing options for University was a bit tricky. I remember feeling angry that British students weren't allowed to choose a wide selection of subjects like they were at American institutions. Being multi-passionate became a headache rather than a plus point, and I can't tell you how many times I changed my mind about what to go for. My heart was telling me 'Music', but I knew that my parents' thoughts on choosing Languages to secure a wider variety of positions after graduating was a sensible one. As a typical Aquarius, I've always been quite good at getting lost in dreams and ideas, but often fall short when grounding my thoughts into reality. The stereotypical 'starving artist' image kept popping into my head again and again, and I knew that it was probably wise to let my head win out over my heart this time.

Looking back however, it was around about this time that I started to get colds and non-stop sore throats. To be honest, I was singing *a lot* in those days, so the sore throats should've come as no surprise. But it was difficult to get my head around the constant colds and flu- I was almost becoming the class joke. My English Literature teacher used to pass me Echinacea tablets under the desk in class, and they seemed to work for a little while when the traditional remedies didn't. I couldn't take any time away from my studies to recover- I was terrified and paranoid about missing something in class that might be in the exam. I couldn't betray my 'A* student' reputation now. I couldn't let my section down at choir, and the netball and athletics team would be down a player. I would gargle and claw my way through the day, and fall into bed completely bunged up, just hoping that I could get enough rest to see me through a few more hours the next day, but the cycle would start all over again.

When I went to get my final exam results from high school, I couldn't open the envelope for about 30 minutes. My Mum had to come into the school building and find me. This had also happened when collecting my previous exam results- I distinctly remember my lovely English teacher opening the brown envelope on my behalf next to my locker because I couldn't bear to do it myself. I was relieved (note I didn't use the word 'happy' or 'joyful') to discover that I had done it- straight As. I had the grades I needed for French at Edinburgh University. My parents and family were over the moon, and I couldn't wait to get started. Edinburgh had always had a special place in my heart from numerous family holidays, and to study there was going to be incredible.

I spoke too soon....

My early excitement however was met with a bit of a fork in the road a few weeks later. Every year, we saved up hard and had a summer holiday somewhere in Europe. It sounds slightly crazy looking back, but we always used to drive from the U.K. At the time though it was great fun and I'm so grateful to have explored some incredible parts of the continent. Being a bit of a linguist, the pressure was always on to order in restaurants and sound like I knew what I was talking about, but I loved the challenge (most of the time) as my knowledge of French and

German improved.

The summer after I finished high school we were lucky enough to go to Tuscany in Italy, but the sweltering heat and overwhelming vibrancy of Tuscan summers got a little bit too much for me. I woke up one morning a little bit later than normal and stumbled into the shower. The last thing I remember was the water vapour quickly moistening the walls of the shower. I woke up in an ambulance, with two very friendly and incredibly relaxed paramedics. I couldn't understand anything of what they were saying and my parents were nowhere to be found. They gestured nonchalantly out of the rear window and I could see my family following in the car, brows creased with worry. To make matters worse, the ambulance driver decided to cheer me up by putting on the siren. I thought it was really sweet of them, but my parents' panic-stricken faces told a very different story.

This was the start of everything for me, but I didn't realise it at the time. What started as a blackout in an Italian bathroom from the heat and lack of breakfast led to multiple blackouts, fainting and panic attacks. I still wasn't back to my old self when we returned home after the holiday. Something had irrevocably shifted. The truth was I was utterly, completely and devastatingly exhausted; wrung-out, hollowed out and spun out, and I *still* had that permanent head cold.

Suddenly University didn't seem so exciting and shiny anymore. I wasn't really looking forward to having to navigate Freshers' Week with a fever, a box of tissues and a feeling like the ground was going to be whipped out from under me at any moment. The whole thing made me feel nauseous. In hindsight, I don't think I realised how panicked my parents were about what had happened in Italy. I'd always been so healthy and athletic, but I knew we might have had a problem on our hands when my Mum suggested counselling.

Going to speak with a counsellor was an incredibly confusing prospect. I didn't really know what was wrong- I didn't have an actual diagnosis and as far as I knew, I was still going to University, so what was I actually here to speak about? Was there some prepared hidden agenda that I was supposed to go along with? It's amazing how the idea of going to speak to a therapist can suddenly make you question everything you know about yourself.

I remember my Mum's face when the session started and she was asked to leave by the counsellor. She looked so worried and tormented, and I know she really wanted to hear my thoughts for herself. In all honesty, I wish I'd been hiding something to make it easier. I wish I'd had a dark, deep secret that warranted counselling, but in truth, I can't even remember the rest of the session. All my energy was in my body, trying to frantically repair the imbalances, trying desperately not to faint or blackout. All I remember is that the sofa and carpet were a murky brown colour, and the harrowing feeling of sheer desperation and sadness afterwards.

I *think* we drove home, but my eyes were masked by floods of ugly sobs. I couldn't even hold my head up. The counsellor had hit something deep within me that I think revealed some hidden resentment and bitterness towards those who had bullied me at school. I was really angry with the counsellor for making me feel like this- I felt blamed, shamed and completely backed into a corner. With hindsight of course, it had nothing to do with the counsellor, rather my own feelings of inadequacy and unworthiness, but I think I was just too young to see it.

"How about taking a gap year and going to University next year?", my Mum offered quietly.

I couldn't believe these words were even coming out of my Mum's mouth- this was so unlike her. I felt relieved for a second, before this rage took over. My intuition told me that my Mum was right, but I couldn't think straight. I was still seething that I'd been made to feel so small by someone I didn't even know minutes earlier.

"No, no, no. That's a stupid idea. What would I do? I'll be fine, I'll be fine", I heard myself say.

That was when my gut feeling popped in, probably the first

time I remember ever feeling it.

"Well, it might be an idea- you've been pretty sick. Let's face it, you're not feeling so great", offered my Mum.

When we returned home, I sat on the floor in my room and stared at my feet. I couldn't take a gap year- *none* of my friends were taking a gap year, we didn't even consider it. I would be so far behind everyone else- what an embarrassment. No, keep going- let's get on with it.

Making it to University

I can barely remember buying things to take up to University with me, a typical rite of passage for a soon-to-be independent young adult, but I know a travel kettle was involved somewhere. On the windy and frustratingly narrow road up to Edinburgh, all I wanted to do was get there. I just wanted to prove myself wrong- I was absolutely fine and there was nothing wrong with me.

I moved into halls and seemed to handle the natural anxiety of it all ok. It completely takes you back to high school, trying to suss out who the cool kids are, and automatically distancing myself from them because I wasn't anywhere near as talented or respectable as they were. I would probably have looked down my nose at me too back then.

I would love to be able to give you a little story or anecdote here that would set the scene of being in such an incredible place as Edinburgh, but I can't. Not because I don't want to, but because I simply don't have any. I remember meeting a few good friends, who tried really hard to understand what was going on with me, but instead of recalling happy times getting to know people in the pub, all I remember is having to turn away invitations. All I remember is trying to muster up enough strength to open my eyes between naps and sleep, and lean on my elbow to pull myself up and text someone to let them know I couldn't make it. Sending a single text message was agonising, not just the piercing pain in my fingers, but also emotionally. Here I was yet again, rejecting a social occasion because I couldn't get out of bed. The only time my phone buzzed was when my family called me.

"I'm fine, I'm fine- everything's great!", I told them.

Until it wasn't.

Stop the Madness

When I tell this story, I'm often paranoid about the fact that people might think I'm being overly dramatic, but I really wish I was exaggerating. It might make the whole experience a little easier to swallow if I were. It's very difficult to describe to others just how distressing this whole experience was, but if you've been there, you might feel your heart jump a little.

After weeks of believing that I was just under the weather and all the excitement of Freshers Week had gotten a little too much for me, over a period of about a week, I suddenly became increasingly worried that I had gone crazy- that I'd totally lost my marbles, and really needed some urgent, psychological help. It was like something had snapped in my brain. Something wasn't right.

Agonising pain in my fingers became searing, incomprehensible pain. My legs were glued to the mattress and even the *thought* of moving a muscle made my head explode with anxiety. What the hell was happening to me?

As any parent would do, my Mum and Dad's initial reaction was just to see how it went- in all probability, it was a bad dose of Freshers' flu. I clung on to this hope as well until I seemed to be getting worse after two weeks. In my comatose state, even *I* realised that having to crawl to the bathroom, a journey that seemed to take the best part of 2 hours, wasn't normal.

One of my old school friends that was in Edinburgh with me took me to see a specialist, but I can't really remember a lot of what happened. I couldn't tell you for the life of me what was said, what was advised or what happened during the appointment. All I can remember is that the bus journey seemed to take forever, and the specialist muttering something about 'Cognitive Behavioural Therapy'.

This is the part where I should be recalling an emotional account about how I felt when I was finally forced to leave University, about having my parents help me pack away my things and feeling embarrassed and humiliated in front of all my friends. But the truth is, I genuinely can't remember any of it. I can't seem to remember any of these events or conversations, or even the next few months after that. All I seem to recollect is having a meeting with one of my tutors (I remember how nervous and anxious I was even just getting there- my head was spinning, and I remember stumbling along the road, just desperate not to bump into anyone I knew or worse, for me to collapse in the street). He was a lovely man and totally understood what was going on. I was given a letter so I could restart my studies in a year's time.

The few months after I came home were spent in another world, a world in which I became a living zombie. While everyone else was awake, I was dead to the world for all of around 21 hours a day.

If you were to ask my parents about this crazy time, they would definitely tell you about the 'blue jumper'. For some reason, I just would not take off this teal-coloured, Topshop jumper while I was sick. I think I wore it more or less constantly for about 6 months, minus my Mum somehow whipping it away when I wasn't looking to wash it. It had buttons on one side of the neck down to the shoulder and fit me perfectly. I think in all honesty I was too exhausted to take it off. My Mum donated it to a charity shop once I got better, but I sometimes wish I had that jumper to look back on that time and all that I went through. It's funny how you remember and recall the little things, even when they don't allude to the happiest of times.

Finally, a name

I remember this scene in the hospital office so vividly, but it was almost as if I wasn't sitting alongside my parents listening to the doctor. I was almost standing behind us all (in my blue jumper) just examining my parents' faces.

When the doctor mentioned the words 'not' and 'leukaemia', my parents both put their head in their hands and wiped their foreheads. I felt like someone had poured boiling and freezing water all over me at the same time. So, what the hell was it?

"There's been very little research done so far on this, but we think Katharine might have Myalgic Encephalomyelitis, otherwise known as M.E.".

I can't really remember the rest of the conversation, but finally, after having undergone every single medical test under the sun, we had something to treat. The doctor would recommend a course of treatment, maybe give me a prescription and give me an estimated recovery time- no problem. But it didn't come and, as I was to learn for myself, it never would. It was recommended that I just ride it out.

Riding something out is tough for anyone. Riding *anything* out when you're a type-A overachiever who's used to having boundless amounts of energy is such a foreign, uncomfortable feeling. I was someone who was just 'on' all the time, and apart from sleep, I never really felt the need to stop and relax (and therein lies the problem). All I could think about was what my high school friends would be doing right now, and how they would react if they found out. So, the swotty, four-eyed teacher's pet had finally been stopped in her tracks. I think a couple of classmates would've been quite pleased to hear that.

I'm not depressed

After that, every day slid away and I was powerless. I would be lying to you if I said that accepting CFS was easy, that literally being a useless shell of a person suited me well. I would be lying if I told you that acceptance washed over me like a warm ocean wave, that I had an awe-inspiring spiritual awakening and suddenly, I just got it. It took me *years* to finally realise that this was how it was going to be for a while, and even then, I wrestled with my illness with everything I had left in me.

I'd also be deceiving you if I said that this section of the book was a breeze for me to write. Even now, I have a huge lump in my throat and feel a little jittery.

The raw, honest truth of it is that I *was* depressed.

Of course I was- how could I *not* have been? I had my whole life and ambitions taken away from me, and was forced to accept some ugly, painful realities that you wouldn't wish on your worst enemy. The whole course of my life as I had known it for 18 years was whipped out from under me and suddenly, it all felt like it belonged to someone else. Well, who was I now? Having friends and family question you, coupled with the fact that there's a huge social stigma attached to CFS anyway, meant that I felt completely alone and uncontrollably angry. Those two emotions in combination are capable of playing havoc with your body *and* mind.

My local village doctor prescribed me antidepressants (Prozac). I remember him sliding the green and white script across the table with a slightly concerned, but insistent look. I took the prescription, but didn't end up getting the tablets. I just couldn't admit to myself that I might need help with this, and to be honest, I didn't feel as dark and fed-up as I thought I *should* be to warrant being on medication for depression. In the end, on my next visit to the doctor, he wrote me out another prescription (I 'accidently' lost the first one). I remember clutching it in my hand and my Dad saying to me, "You know, I have to take medication for my cholesterol. Maybe you could take something for a little while to level everything out a bit." After looking in my Dad's eyes and seeing how much he cared, I decided to get the tablets from the pharmacy.

I didn't stay on the antidepressants for very long though. I think I lasted about 3 months before coming off them. I felt nauseous taking them and intuitively knew that this was not the right thing for my body. Some people might say that I should have stuck with them for longer, but I just couldn't bring myself to take them anymore. It wasn't me.

You see, I always knew that mine wasn't a deep, dark depression. It just felt kind of....sticky. A viscous substance that I couldn't quite get off my hands or out of my head. We shouldn't really compare someone else's experience of depression with our own, but some part of me needed to cling on to that element of separation. I never had thoughts about ending my life or harming myself in any way and I didn't seek counselling for the very same reasons. I revisited the same doctor about every 2-3 weeks while I was at home, just hoping that some new information had come to light, but it never came. I remember really resenting my doctor, but how could I be angry at him when no-one else seemed to have the answers either?

Frankly, for about 3 dark months, I think I was in absolute

shock. I barely spoke to anyone. It's only since fully recovering that I've become interested in the nature of shock and trauma, and how long it takes for our brain to catch up with our body. I was disturbed at how different my life was before my diagnosis to how it was now and I just couldn't get my head around the disparity in energy levels and my general appetite for life. This is the main reason why I believe I was more depressed than I admitted to be at the time- I had no desire to do anything. I was completely apathetic. Even when I was making progress, having a shower was just too much effort, not necessarily because I didn't have the energy, but because I couldn't see the point of it. I wasn't able to go out of the house and my family had seen me in worse states, so why bother? When someone asked me how I was, I didn't see the use in telling them- I was just admitting to myself what I already knew, and which they intuitively knew as well- that nothing had changed (in fact I felt worse) and I was still feeling beyond shitty. More shitty than I ever thought it was possible for someone to feel. I felt like a slug who was crawling along on wet ground beneath everyone else, and what little I had left of my self esteem had totally vanished.

Eventually, I didn't want to fight anymore, so for the sake of my family (they didn't deserve my anger), I started forcing myself to respond even though I didn't want to. I started accepting their help when everything inside of me told me not to bother. I let them bundle me into the car and take me to the supermarket- my weekly trip out- even though my face was tripping me up, I looked a sight and I could barely say a word because of brain fog. It was only when I regularly forced myself into these incredibly uncomfortable situations that I realised my perspective was changing. Sometimes even being in a supermarket surrounded by strangers rummaging around in the frozen food section can bring you a surreal sense of community and belonging.

Weren't we all just rummaging around in the frozen food section?

CHAPTER 3
IS THIS REALLY HAPPENING?

The months after my diagnosis were a bit of a blur. I still had terrible brain fog, which was especially bad in the morning just after waking. It felt like my eyelids were constantly trying to slam shut, forcing me back to sleep, but ever the stubborn one, I fought to keep them wide open.

My sleeping patterns were still absolutely non-existent. It's incredibly ironic that an illness whose main symptom is overwhelming tiredness can cause such incredible insomnia, yet another cruel twist for CFS sufferers. I remember waking up well after my parents had left for work, at around 11.30am, spending the afternoon dozing in bed (shutting my eyes for what felt like 5 seconds before realising that 3 hours had passed) and then being wide-awake from about 9pm to 4.30am (the computer game, Mah-jong, became my best friend. Matching tiles up on a screen was all that my little brain could handle, and it was the only thing I could do which involved not waking anybody else up in the house.) My parents would often peek into the study to check I was ok, but they soon accepted that this thing would just have to ride itself out (those words again). The once weekly walk around the supermarket was, begrudgingly, still happening.

About 5 months after I arrived home, my sleeping patterns gradually started to reorganise themselves. I was waking up at around noon and sleeping at 2am- not perfect, but it was progress. It was at around this point that my Mum ventured that they needed a hand in the photocopying room at school and it might be a good way to get me up on my feet again, so to speak. Of course, I point-blank refused for weeks. How could I stand up and use a photocopier all day when standing up to brush my teeth was nearly impossible? With hindsight my Mum must've pulled a lot of strings to get this opportunity for me. Sometimes all we can see when we're sick is people trying to interfere in what's going on and trying to make our lives harder, when really they're just trying to show us that they care about us. I eventually gave in, but I wasn't happy about it and I knew that physically, I probably wouldn't be able to manage it anyway. I wasn't motivated by getting paid either, because saving up to go shopping seemed completely pointless when I couldn't stand to be anywhere near crowds.

As it turned out (and believe me, at the time I did everything in my power to make it difficult for myself), the job at my Mum's school 2 days a week was one of the best things that could have happened for me. Mum drove me there and back, the photocopy room was quiet with minimal social interaction (great for brain foggy days), and if I needed a little time out, the ladies I worked with were incredibly understanding. I found the repetitive nature of photocopying quite soothing and enjoyed not having to deal with unexpected stress. This is not to say that I recommend diving into a job straight away, but it made me feel as though there was life outside my bedroom, that people aside from my family were genuinely interested in how I was and more importantly, that there were more things to think about in the world than being ill or the possibility of becoming sicker overnight. Even though I often found it excruciatingly painful to wake up some days and worked with acute pain in my hands (one of my relapse triggers), I would get home at the end of the day, dive back under the duvet and know that I had achieved something.

Eventually, I was able to move up to 3 days a week and take on more responsibilities, such as working on the reception desk. I was going to add in a sentence here about how proud I was of myself for doing this and I was, but some days my ego jumped in the way and the shame was crushing. I used to be a high-flying student and now I was having trouble picking up the phone and remembering my own name. If I had a bad evening or made myself anxious before going to work, my symptoms always got worse. I remember looking at the students who were just finishing school and leaving to go to University, and wanting so badly to be them- so full of energy and optimism. I couldn't help but make comparisons and jump between who I was in the past and who I seemed to be now. Even though my family were pleased with my progress, I was my own worst enemy, and thought that they were just trying to appease me, that they didn't really mean it. In my mind, I was practically a toddler again, needing help from others and not yet capable of standing on my own two feet.

University- Round Two

After 3 months of part-time work, I had to inform my University about whether I would be returning to study or not. This was it, sink or swim. I knew that they wouldn't keep my place open for another year, so in many ways the decision had already been made- it was out of my hands.

It was at the end of September when I took up my place at Edinburgh University again. A part of me couldn't wait to leave home, but another part of me knew that it was going to be more difficult than I thought. I knew that lectures were going to be strenuous and that having to explain to people why (yet again) I might not be able to join in Freshers activities wasn't something I was looking forward to. The apprehension was overwhelming and truth be told, I was petrified. If there's anything my little job at Mum's school had taught me though, it's that we should always allow for the element of surprise. If I ended up at home again, so be it. Maybe I would just have to accept that University might be too much for me altogether.

This time however, we decided on self-catering University flats which were about a 15 minute walk (up a very steep hill) to my lecture theatres and the Languages building. I remember the look on my parents' faces when they gave me the 'daughter is going to University' look for the second time, but there was more concern in their eyes this time around, just hoping that I would be well enough to get the most out of it.

My flatmates were lovely and first year lectures weren't as terrifying as I thought they were going to be. I was pleased to discover that I could still remember elements of my studies from school and I hadn't lost it all in the brain fog. However, I had to miss a lot of the tutorials, because they started at around 9am or 10am, which was a little bit much. I hadn't completely broken my sleeping patterns and was still slightly nocturnal, listening to the students on the area known as the Cowgate below me at 2am, dropping glass bottles, shouting drunken slurs and singing off-key. This became my 'daily' routine, and my flatmates also seemed to have developed a liking for partying into the wee small hours, so all was well...until, yet again, it wasn't.

Having got through my first year not having to sit any French exams because of a high grade average (I still can't tell you how I managed that), my flatmates told me that they weren't inviting me to find a flat with them for second year. They said that we were too different and that they just couldn't cope with me being ill, even though I barely saw them and spent a lot of time in bed (which was probably the issue). It was difficult not to be upset, especially as I knew it'd be complicated to find someone who would be ok putting up with my illness. There were no hard feelings, but I could remember the way it felt to be rejected, just like being in school again.

Very, *very* luckily, a few days later, a friend who I had met when I first started University offered a room to me for my second year. It was a little bit further out of town, but to be honest, I was still struggling with juggling my illness and all the intense pressure of studying, so being away from the rest of the students turned out to be a real bonus. I had always been extra-sensitive to sounds and noise, and the area we were staying in was perfect. The nightlife wasn't jumping, but then again, who was I kidding?

It was around this time that I started to get severe migraines for the first time in my life. You'd think I would've struggled with these a lot more when I was first diagnosed, but they didn't really affect me. I ended up missing hours of Italian tutorials as a result (I'd picked it up as an extra language), and absolutely scraped the exam. I loved Italian, but learning another language completely from scratch with brain fog and a body that felt like it could crumble at any minute maybe wasn't such a great move.

When you're studying a Languages degree, it's normally obligatory to spend your third year in the country whose language you're learning, either studying at a University or working, so I decided to apply to become an English Language teaching assistant. I would get paid and was especially reassured to find out that I would be living within the school grounds. It couldn't have been better.

You've got to be kidding, right?

However, this feeling of freedom was short-lived. Getting struck down with serious glandular fever about a month before I was due to leave was just what I needed. A lot of people become ill with CFS after having glandular fever, so why was I in for the reverse double-whammy? I also became jaundiced meaning that my skin started turning a rather peculiar shade of yellow. At the time, I was trying a new type of moisturiser with fake tan in it, which was all the rage. But I knew something wasn't quite right when my Brother suggested maybe laying off the moisturiser, only for me to tell him that I hadn't used it in weeks. I was drinking gallons of water and all I seemed to be able to eat was ice cream. My parents had to return from a week away, and I was rushed into hospital because my liver was inflamed.

The only thing I had to cling on to during my time in hospital were two things: the prospect of heading to France in a few weeks' time and the new Harry Potter book. I didn't even really think about CFS- I think I just put glandular fever down to the fact that I normally became sick with whatever was going around at the time (I'm sure if you've got CFS, you'll know what I mean). I think we mentioned something about it to the hospital when I was admitted, but it didn't really change anything. Suddenly, my year abroad was in jeopardy, and if I didn't make it to France, I would get a general Bachelor's degree instead of a Master's degree. I remember quite clearly telling my parents, "I am going to France if I have to drag my bed with me." I don't think I realised how sick I was, but somehow, I made it to France. I couldn't stop now- it was too much of an opportunity.

Vive la France

France was a huge turning point in my life. I was so glad that I ended up in a small village instead of a big city. The students and staff at the school I was teaching at were great, and the teaching load was surprisingly manageable. There was even a teachers strike about 3 months in and we didn't work for 2 months. It was only around 2 hours to get to Paris by train, and it really helped me to pace myself and establish a routine of resting and self-care. It's incredible what happens when you're given an opportunity to reset and look at things from a different perspective, but honestly, after what I went through during the summer, I really didn't think I'd be there.

However, this is not to say it was always straightforward. I became quite homesick just after I started, which, when you're exclusively communicating in another language, can make things even more painful. I also found myself having blood tests done at the doctors, as I was overwhelmingly tired, but all of a sudden and in the morning about an hour or two after waking up. Even snacking and regulating my eating didn't help. Before one of the members of my department drove me to the doctors, I remember telling myself that they wouldn't find anything, and I was right- they couldn't find anything in my blood tests. You can become familiar with this feeling a lot of the time when you have CFS. You almost want to tell them not to bother in the first place. In true French style, I was told to take a few days off and eat lots of croissants (seriously!). Well, when in France..!

It took me a long time to ride out that little wobble, and unusually, at the time, the word 'relapse' didn't even enter my head. It was as though being in another country completely wiped away any relationship I had to the illness. I was just a little tired and we were going through a cold winter- no big deal. Magnesium tablets were the supplement 'du jour', so I took those for a while as prescribed by the doctor, and they still form a regular part of my wellness routine today.

I led a very simple life in France, but it was incredibly freeing- weekend markets and trips on the train, cheap cinemas ticket and winter walks through the vineyards. After severe bouts of homesickness while I was settling in, suddenly I was going to have to return to the U.K., and I really didn't want to.

After returning from France, I felt revived, but also as though I'd drifted away from a lot of my friends who didn't have to spend a year abroad as part of their degrees. A lot can happen in a year and, as many of you can relate to, it's often difficult to put into words all of the experiences you've had in your life over the space of nearly a year. I grew apart from many people, but I think because this had happened earlier in my life as part of my diagnosis, I didn't take it as badly as I think many others would've done. Rather than dwelling on the fact that I seemed to be starting from zero again, I took this as a sign that new friends and relationships would be coming into my life. They did, but only when my incredible, final year of University schedule allowed them to.

The Final Push, and a Little Surprise

I remember looking at my fourth year French reading list and not knowing what had hit me. I had 4 literature modules to prepare for, and they each consisted of around 7 texts. In French. 28 books to annotate, learn the historical background and context of and be asked extended essay questions about. I think if I'd been presented with this reading list in first or second year after restarting, I probably would've relapsed out of sheer panic and maybe have had to drop out again. But something happened to me in France- I really learned to prioritise taking time out just for me and to focus on priorities. Being in a tiny village definitely had its advantages, and with hindsight, I knew I'd been sent there for a reason. Suddenly this huge reading list didn't seem so terrible- I knew I had no choice but to get on with it.

The Universe also decided to throw a bit of a spanner in the works about 3 weeks before my final exams. My friend had been in the pub all afternoon and was screaming at me down the phone to come and join her at a party around the corner from my flat (a 'revision break', as she put it.)

The first person I saw as we opened the door to the party was a guy called Frazer and something happened in that moment. To cut a very long (but kind of cute!) story short, a party I didn't want to be at became a party I didn't want to leave. In an effort to keep myself sane during my finals, I was determined to act cool, saying that I 'didn't have time' for a relationship, but I couldn't do it. It was beyond me. I could easily have panicked and ignored what was happening with Frazer, but I just couldn't.

However, I *did* get slightly panicked at the thought of my final exams. It had all been going pretty well health-wise during the year, but what if I suddenly relapsed the week before, or what if I sat one exam, but the stress and fatigue made it impossible to sit the rest of them? I know exams are taxing for most people, but the (imaginary) possibility of deteriorating health was more stressful than any medieval French text ever would be. I knew that I needed to ask for help and I have to say, I was incredibly embarrassed and almost ashamed to request to be referred to the University's Disability office. Even though I knew I probably should've asked for support in first year, the thought only occurred to me in my final few weeks of term. I just knew that doing my exam in a separate room with lots of others who were given extra time might just take the edge off my stress a little bit. I truly believe that if I hadn't done it, I might not have made it to the end of my exams. I had nine, 3-hour whoppers, and I felt like I'd been hit by a brick when I finished the last one. I remember meeting Frazer (now my husband) after my final one and stumbling down the brown, shiny corridor to meet him, realising that not only had I finished my exams and led a relatively 'normal' existence for the last year, but I'd also somehow managed to get a degree. I couldn't believe it. I couldn't believe that that same person who had spent a whole year in bed in absolute disbelief, detachment, pain and discomfort, had somehow managed to finish University.

I'm incredibly lucky that I was functioning at about 80% when I met Frazer. I was able to go out on dates, go to parties *and* complete all of my University exams. Looking back on it, it was all a bit of a whirlwind- I was constantly worried that I'd wake up one morning and feel those all-too-familiar aches and pains and would have to just go back to square one. But I'm pleased (and slightly baffled) to say that that didn't happen.

CHAPTER 4
MOVING ON UP

I was happy to spend that summer at home and return to Edinburgh for my graduation ceremony. Michael Palin, one of my favourite people, was giving a speech and I really felt like I belonged in that space with all of the other successful graduates.

I decided for my next step to dive into my High School Teacher Training at Durham University, the University of my hometown, and to stay with my parents while I was studying. I have to be completely frank and say that it was a 'let's see what happens' decision. I knew I didn't want a typical desk job or to be in the corporate world, so teaching seemed like a good option. One of my school friends had previously done the same course at Durham and told me it would be infinitely more stressful than my final year at Edinburgh. I couldn't believe it would be more hellish than that, but I was completely wrong. If anyone out there has done teacher training or knows somebody who has, you'll know that you will be pushed to your absolute limits. To a lot of people on the outside, teaching is just a cushy, little 9am-3pm job, but the reality would shock a lot of people.

I think by this stage, I believed that the worst was behind me with CFS. I was still taking a lot of 'just in case' vitamins and supplements and shunning a lot of social invitations (again, 'just in case'), but I had to change my focus and attention to completing my course, CFS or no CFS.

Teacher training in the UK is completed in a year, and while it might seem as though that's all it takes to hone your skills, you end up squeezing every single minute out of that year. We had lectures and tutorials back-to-back, along with 2 blocks of time spent in a 'real' school on a reduced teaching timetable. My first placement was 4 weeks long and this was when my perfectionist self really rose up and hit me between the eyes. Every single aspect of my lesson had to be perfect. If a student acted up or an activity didn't go the way I thought it would, I would beat myself up about it for days afterwards. Little did I know how wasteful this energy would be in the long-run, especially when you've got a full teaching load, as well as numerous other school-based responsibilities.

Just when I could see the light at the end of the placement, all my stress and anxiety caught up with me, and I got really bad flu. It was winter in the UK and to be honest, I didn't draw any link between being out-of-my-mind stressed at work to being sick. Everyone got sick in winter, didn't they? I remember being absolutely baffled at my then Head of Department who went swimming every evening on her way home from school to relax after a frantic day. How could she afford the time? How could she be so utterly chilled out? I learned in hindsight that she was doing what I now know is crucial to not just recovery, but life in general. In the words of the inimitable Dale Carnegie, "Rest before you get tired." Still, in my naivety, I couldn't fathom how or why my mentor felt the need to care for herself so unashamedly and on a daily basis without fail. Didn't she have work to do?

The Christmas holidays were spent writing essays. Even on the afternoon of Christmas Day (yep, I was that far over the line), I had a spare hour while everyone was dozing off to make some leeway on my Master's essay about bullying, a topic very close to my heart for reasons you read about earlier. Rather than comment on how rude I was being or whether it might be a good idea just to give it a rest for a day, my parents just left me. They knew that I'd work whether they insisted I had a day off or not.

For my second, longer placement, I had more of the same, but this time instead of becoming sick, my stress and anxiety played out in a different way. Because I was so stressed and so keen to make sure that all the students thought I was wonderful (an affliction a lot of teachers have, whether they'll admit to it or not), nutrition and the amount I was eating really fell by the wayside. Breakfast was taken care of, as my Grandparents who I was staying with for this placement, insisted that I sat down with them and had a good breakfast, bless them. All the other bits in between however weren't as easy. Lunch, if I remembered to grab something at all, was half a piece of bread, a few crackers or a mug of instant soup. No wonder I was seeing stars after my last lesson of the day. I had absolutely no sense of what it meant to nourish yourself or respect your body's need for natural (non-synthetic) nutrition. I managed to convince myself that the act of sitting down, chilling out and eating was a total waste of time when I could be maximising my multi-tasking time. I always managed to eat *something*, but I turned into someone who definitely eats for fuel, rather than for any kind of enjoyment, pleasure or self-respect.

Moving to London?

After passing my teacher training alive, mostly unscathed and with no more illnesses or sniffles to write home about, Frazer and I decided to take a big leap and move to London.

This is where things took a turn for me, and not in a good way. I suddenly realised, as I lumped boxes and torn carrier bags into my new flat-share, that I always said I was never going to move to London and I always said I was never going to be a teacher. Here I was, fulfilling both prophecies in the blink of an eye. What in the world was going on?

I deliberately chose a house about a 20-minute walk away from school as I knew my first year of teaching with a full timetable was going to be hectic to say the least. Frazer found a house on the other side of London and I spent most weekends over there (if only to avoid students bumping into me in the supermarket and attempting to rifle through my shopping basket). In all honesty, this was the best thing we could have done at this stage in our relationship, as I was a total nightmare and pretty much, as during my teacher training, worked solidly from the second I got home to the moment I decided to try and do something called 'sleep'.

For the 2 years after I started teaching, I would wake up during the night every hour, on the hour, which of course followed that even getting to sleep in the first place was almost an impossibility. It was almost the complete polar opposite of my days of being severely affected by M.E. when I could barely yank my eyelids open. I had this big alarm clock, which would angrily spit out the time at me in red whenever I glanced at it. Even at the weekends, this 'wired' feeling persisted, as I spent every Sunday travelling back from Frazer's flat before jumping into school work again. I even felt bad for sitting 'doing nothing' on the tube on the way home or stopping off to buy groceries- any moment spent not doing school work seemed to pull me further and further into the pits of being a rubbish teacher, and therefore a rubbish human being.

Even as I'm writing this, I have to laugh at myself and wonder what I was trying to prove, and what had gotten into me back then. You've probably realised by now that all this perfectionism covered up my incredible fear of not being good enough. I think being sick for so long distorts your view of the world slightly and makes you believe that you're not entitled to fun, that any opportunity you have to relax and enjoy yourself is probably going to end up with you being in bed or relapsing, so what's the point? This might sound a little sombre, but I'm sure I'm not the only one who carries this around with them from some kind of major illness or physical crash. It's almost as if you don't trust your body not to betray you again- the fear of 'what if' seems to always threaten what we're doing or want to do in the world.

Again, right on cue, about 8 weeks into teaching and at more-or-less the same time it happened the year before, I got the flu, but it was worse this time. It was at this stage that I started to think that there might be more to this episode than just the frosty weather. This time however, I had a whole timetable, students and colleagues to consider, and in true type-A personality style, I carried on teaching until I was at death's door and ended up having to take a week off. In the grand scheme of things, a week isn't that long and I couldn't help it, but I felt the need to constantly apologise for being absent. My more-experienced colleagues however didn't really understand why I was apologising so much, but looking back, I think I was almost apologising to myself for letting myself down. The more I said sorry, the more I felt I was moving towards a blinding realisation that I wasn't worthy of love. I wasn't worthy of free time at the weekends or, shock horror, during the week. I would constantly check my work emails when I was tucked up and feverish in bed, hoping somehow that the students and staff knew that I was still serious and dedicated to my work, that I was still entirely perfect and irreplaceable even though I wasn't physically there.

This frantic daily routine continued for months, and well into the next year- flinging myself from one lesson to the next, still not eating very well, saying 'yes' to everyone and everything in the hope that people would think I was good at my job and not managing to grab more than two hours of sleep in succession.

I needed a bit of a kick, a wake-up call. If I was going to pin-point another event that would completely define where I am today and the insights that have revealed themselves to me thick and fast, this would be it, and ironically, it had nothing to do with M.E.

CHAPTER 5
TAKING A TUMBLE

It had snowed so heavily in London one night during the second year of teaching that the Underground system was completely off. The roads were in total chaos and our school had closed for the day. Gazing at the thick blanket of white out my bedroom window, I had a gut feeling that I shouldn't be moving a muscle (an interesting choice of phrase, as we're just about to find out!) I would have some breakfast and maybe catch up on some schoolwork. However, a few of the members of my department had gone into work, so I thought it best that I went in too, even though the students weren't there. The one thing I now realise is that a lot of colleagues had cars, but I didn't.

So, a walk that would normally take 20 minutes took me close to an hour in knee-deep snow. Just as I thought I'd reached the home stretch, I started to get complacent, and I fell.

I fell really, really badly. I fell so badly that a bus driver who'd been passing the bus stop I fell by jumped off the bus to check that I was ok, as did about 20 of his passengers. The driver hoisted me up to sit on one of those unfathomably thin benches you find in bus shelters as I tried to stop my ugly sobbing. I insisted that I was ok after my 'Tom and Jerry' fall and that I didn't need an ambulance. After I pulled myself together from the shock, I managed to drag myself the 50 metres or so into school and went straight into the Nurse's office to lie down. I can still remember how much pain I was in, and it makes me feel sick to my stomach.

I felt like a total idiot. I had completely ignored my intuition and got myself into a huge mess. I was driven to the Doctor's surgery and told that I would have to take three days off school. I was kind of getting the hang of this 'listening to advice' thing, so I did what I was told. However, a week later, I was still in absolute agony, but the pain had moved from the base of my spine to my hip. Convincing myself that it was probably just a bit of residual pain, I kept on going, teaching with a limp on a crutch and wincing every time I tried to carry something or write on the board- I was a total mess. I guess I wasn't as good at listening to advice as I thought I was.

After a colleague insisted on taking me to the hospital, it turns out that I'd really hurt myself. I had a probable hairline fracture in my pelvis and the muscles around my hip were twisted. The pain was now moving up into my back and neck, and I couldn't bear anyone touching me.

After about three weeks of me carrying on working like nothing had happened, I woke up one morning and couldn't move. My fingers, toes, pelvis, arms and fingertips were glued to the mattress and I was in total agony. When had I experienced this before? It felt familiar. Then it dawned on me that I was going through the exact same physical sensations in my body as when I was experiencing my most severe M.E. symptoms at University. This time however, I was alert- my mind was on overdrive. In some ways, when we're so sick with M.E., it's a blessing in disguise that our brain isn't as awake as we'd like it to be, otherwise we'd drive ourselves crazy. This is what was happening to me. Imagine the combination of my controlling, perfectionist personality on overdrive with the severe pain and bodily discomfort of M.E. I would have laughed out loud at the irony of it all if I wasn't in complete and utter agony.

Once again, the first thing I thought about was school and my colleagues. I'm not sure what it is about M.E. that turns us into people who are only concerned that others are ok when we're clearly not coping ourselves. Most other people would take their doctor's advice and stay away from work or physical activity, but I had learned the hard way that my way was not the highway. Even though I knew I was going to be away for a while, I persisted in emailing my colleagues, asking if they needed anything and constantly worrying morning, noon and night about how my classes were doing. Gradually though (very gradually), as they reassured me, I started to worry less about school and worry more about what the hell was going on with me.

Every night, Frazer spoke with me about needing to take care of myself and that school would cope without me. He must've realised that he wasn't quite getting through to me when I was still trying to interfere with how things were going at work and pushing myself physically to the point of relapse. Very gradually, he stopped giving me advice- what was the point when I wasn't listening anyway?

I knew that something had to change. I had zero quality of life. Was it the job or was it me? Even at the weekend, I constantly thought about the huge pile of work I had to do the week afterwards, and it was truly never ending. I could always justify the work I was doing for the greater good, so found myself perpetually working, just so that one student might get a slightly higher mark than they did the last time. I was 100% convinced that making yourself sick and ignoring doctor's advice meant that I must've been a dedicated teacher.

If I returned to school for a third year, I knew deep down

that I wouldn't be able to cope with a full teaching load, not for the foreseeable future. Although my M.E. symptoms had flared up slightly and I still wasn't sleeping well, it was my back and neck that were causing me the greatest problems. I took a long hard look at the next academic year, but knew that I couldn't go the way I had been going. Even when I panicked about money and what lay ahead, I knew I had no other option.

A Change in Approach

It was actually a taxi service that got me to see the other side of the story. I used to go to physio once a week , and I would call our local taxi service to get me to the surgery, as I couldn't walk there myself. I think the guy on the end of the phone took pity on me, and always recognised my voice straightaway. He was so calm and kind, asking how everything was going and if my pain was improving. There was always something in his voice that told that whatever happened, I'd be ok.

It was about this time, after getting fed up of relapses and always pushing myself that little bit too far that I started experimenting with halving my expectations. It took me a long, *long* time to get this one and accept it as an effective part of my recovery.

Because we have such high expectations for ourselves and

most of us are striving to way beyond what our body is capable of when we're ill, we want to go all out. I wasn't happy to just get out of the house and walk up the road. I wanted to get out the house, walk up the road, do a load of shopping (always more than I could carry) and then take the scenic route back home because I was just so happy to be out of the house. I used to psyche myself up for it the day before, but on waking just knew that what I'd wanted for myself wasn't going to happen.

Halving my expectations or halving the journey I had envisaged for myself didn't feel right at the beginning and that's because my ego was telling me that I should be capable of more- "What's the matter with you? You can only walk half a block? You used to be an athlete! What a lemon!". I guarantee that you *will* hear this voice on a loop, just as I did, and all you can do is tell it, very kindly, to mind its own business. I was always constantly on the lookout for this voice, as it always tried to get in the way of what I'd set out for myself. I have to be honest and say that I did listen to it sometimes- it absolutely screamed at me- but I became increasingly aware of this fear and deep knowing in my stomach.

If I wanted to walk two blocks, I'd walk one block and come back home. I know, pathetic, right? Wrong, my dear. I had gotten to where I wanted to be and back and I didn't feel as though I was going to collapse on the sofa in a big mess for a month. Sometimes, I didn't feel as though I'd achieved anything, but I had to get over it- I really, *really* had to.

I repeated this several times and only then did I try and go a bit further. Again, I was always on the look out for my ego voice, which tried to push and push and push me. I had to lead with my soul voice, that loving voice that always speaks to us so kindly when we're willing to listen.

Deciding to give up high school teaching, the career that I had trained intensively for, was incredibly difficult, but looking back, it was an amazing exercise in letting go. Although I felt like a failure and that I would never be able to recover from the shame I felt at the time (it still makes me wince to this day), it was the best thing I could've done. I had to move forward because there was no alternative. The only way was onward and it was all I could do not to turn round and look behind me.

For the next few months, I decided to tutor high school students after school, but I was still recovering from the strain I'd put my body under. Because I tended to work in the early evenings, I was lucky enough to be able to lie in, so if I was a little brain fogged or achy, I could still work later in the evening. The number of clients I took on increased, and I was gradually able to regain some kind of life outside the restrictions my health placed upon me.

I make it sound pretty easy, but if you're going through any kind of physical discomfort, you'll know that there's always more to a recovery story than meets the eye. Although I was feeling grateful and relieved that I was managing to create a career that suited me, I still wasn't completely 'there' yet. I was a complete hypochondriac, and would raid the local chemist or supermarket aisle for every vitamin and supplement under the sun. My bag was full of paracetamol, throat sweets and glucose tablets, which I tended to chew on if I was feeling panicked or a little wobbly (whether I really needed them or not). As long as I carried these around in my bag, I felt safe and able to nip any oncoming illness in the bud. What I only came to realise later on however was that I every time I glanced into my bag, I was telling my body that it was sick. I was inviting illness into my life. The more my brain and body received this message, the more I became susceptible to every single cold and flu bug going. Winter in the U.K. can be quite unforgiving, but I was sick every winter, no exceptions. I had *told* my body that it was in bad shape and that my immune system was weak; therefore, I just *had* to be sick. This didn't just happen in winter though- spring, autumn and summer were fair game as well. If I thought my health was *too* good and things were progressing *too* well, I would fill my 'sickness' void, but telling my body that it *was* too good to be true, and it worked every time. My body started displaying symptoms within hours.

I was just a sick person and I had to get used to it. I was always going to be like this.

Around 3 months into tutoring, with my health neither improving nor getting worse, my husband and I realised that we really needed a change. We had both started our careers in London, but often felt stuck in such a huge city. It had its fun moments, but we decided that we badly needed to move. We also knew instinctively that we couldn't stay in the U.K.- we craved a break and a sprinkling of adventure. We thought about Spain, but the language would've held us back a little bit. We then moved on to other English-speaking countries and found ourselves looking at flights to Australia.

The rest, as they say, is history, but booking those one-way flights to Australia means more to me now than I ever thought it would then.

CHAPTER 6
A CHANGE OF SCENERY

I knew as soon as we set foot in Australia that something was changing in our lives. We travelled around South-East Asia for a few months and my body seemed to have balanced itself out a little. I was sleeping (what a novelty!), and my aches and pains were few and far between, even when carrying a backpack twice my size. Even though we'd booked a one-way ticket to Australia and had no idea what was in store for us, I never for a second thought about what might happen if it didn't work out. All I knew was that this incredible country which we still call our home would impact us in a major way. To be honest, flying over Sydney Harbour and seeing the Opera House on a gloriously sunny day would make anyone pack their bags.

We both found 'career' jobs in Sydney and started working away. I was absolutely desperate to change careers in the process of moving countries, but found myself teaching English to international students. Even though I had originally applied to do student administration because I wasn't 100% sure I was ready to stand up all day and teach, I took this as a sign that I was good to go. The teaching schedule was manageable- we finished teaching at 1pm, so if I was having a bad day, I was able to just head home and rest. The nature of teaching is very spontaneous and some days require more of you than others, so it was sometimes difficult to predict how much energy I'd have. But to my surprise, I was virtually symptom-free, even while working.

I always felt as though I was looking over my shoulder though. In a similar way to filling my bag with paracetamol and throat sweets (just in case), I think psychologically I was almost waiting for something terrible to happen. I had to explore this 'darkness' a little more and I became incredibly curious as to the journey from bedridden to being able to stand up and teach day in, day out. Had the move to Australia changed me? Was the change of scenery all that was needed? Surely there was more to all this than just jumping on a plane. I hadn't told anybody at work that I'd been sick. I carried it round with me like a shameful, dirty secret, even though I had absolutely nothing to be ashamed of. Sometimes fear of being stigmatised makes us even more unlikely to share our vulnerabilities with others.

As Brené Brown says in her fabulous book, 'The Gifts of

Imperfection':

"Owning our story can be hard but not nearly as difficult as spending our lives running from it. Embracing our vulnerabilities is risky but not nearly as dangerous as giving up on love and belonging and joy—the experiences that make us the most vulnerable. Only when we are brave enough to explore the darkness will we discover the infinite power of our light."

I realised within a few months of being in Australia that I hadn't owned my story yet. I seemed to have just woken up from a long, drawn-out trance and felt like I'd been spat out the other side. I needed someone to help me make sense of what had been happening to my body over the last 10 years and to help me go that extra 10%. I was so close to a full recovery, but I knew that psychologically, I was letting memories and scars from the past knock me down and affect my present.

It was around this time, as with so many others stories in which people need to reclaim their health, that Louise Hay's ground-breaking book, 'You Can Heal Your Life', fell off the shelf one afternoon. As the book dragged me to the counter, I began to worry about what others would think of me reading this book- would the cashier think I was a complete weirdo? Was I really that broken? (Weren't self-help books a little bit wet and 'woo woo'?)

"Excellent choice", said the cashier, as I nudged the book

over to him. It seemed as though someone had been listening in to my thoughts. I knew that if I was scared of buying a book, I had a long way to go.

The most intriguing part about Louise Hay's book for me is the section at the back in which she lists illnesses and diseases, suggests reasons why we might be experiencing these symptoms and gives an accompanying affirmation to change the way we think about our situation. Although I approached the 'fatigue' section with absolute trepidation, Louise's words jumped out at me as if covered in glitter, dancing and screaming my name:

"Resistance, boredom. Lack of love for what one does."

To give me an extra slap in the chops, the 'chronic disease' section read:

"A refusal to change. Fear of the future. Not feeling safe."

I couldn't believe how true these words were for me. After not studying Music, all I had ever known in my young adult life, and not allowing myself to recover fully from all of those colds and flus I had in my last two years of high school, I was refusing to change. I couldn't envisage who I was without my past successes and academic achievements. I was a complete shell, and definitely didn't feel safe or confident in what the future held. I was tired of living a life that I believed wasn't meant for me, and I resisted any alternative with every cell in my body.

Reading this whole section at the back of Louise Hay's

book was like having the wind taken out of you suddenly-completely upsetting, almost hurtful, but also knowing that there was some grain of truth to what was in front of me. I didn't really know what to do with this new information that had been gifted to me, but it did not leave me. I thought about it in the shower, before I went to bed, and during the night when it woke me up at 3 o'clock in the morning. Who was I without CFS? I thought that I *had* built a life that I loved, so why was I still clinging on to my past, stubbornly refusing to change?

The next book that seemed to find me almost immediately after I'd finished 'You Can Heal Your Life' was Caroline Myss', 'Anatomy of the Spirit'. The title scared the life out of me, and I had no idea why I was supposed to read this book. What would my parents say if they knew I was reading a 'spiritual' book? This was so far removed from anything I'd ever been interested in reading before. I kept thumbing the cover, putting off starting it until I was ready. But would I ever be ready?

Ever since finishing the book, Caroline Myss is probably the author whose work I follow the most. Some people aren't always ready to hear her teachings, but her words struck me in just the right place and at *exactly* the right time. I honestly don't know where I'd be today if I hadn't picked up that book, and I'm so incredibly grateful to her.

I realised while reading that I had been carrying Chronic Fatigue Syndrome and Chronic Illness with me for a lot longer than I really needed to. Although it was painful to admit this at the time, being sick can sometimes bring some positives with it. Ultimately, I think that spending every day in bed made me feel safe- it was easier just to play small and avoid any possible dramas. My diagnosis gave me time out from the rest of the world to reset and hide. I didn't want anything to do with my life if I couldn't be the person I had been. I wasn't willing to adapt or move on and my body gave me exactly what I was looking for. Being sick also allowed other people to look after me, and as terrifying as this is to admit, I think I really wanted my parents to know how angry I was that I hadn't followed my heart. This wasn't really anything to do with them, but often we seek approval and crave love from those closest to us. It was really myself that I was furiously angry at, and I hadn't released any of this anger during my diagnosis, so was carrying it with me. It's traditionally believed that problems of the liver are rooted in anger issues, and my time spent in hospital with glandular fever and jaundice was the outward manifestation of this. Even though I'd returned to University and had been studying French, getting sick just before going to France was one, final "this shouldn't be happening to me!". I still couldn't bring myself to accept that things hadn't turned out the way I planned and I was clinging on to this reality for dear life.

I'd been hanging on to the illness because I didn't really want to change. It had become inseparable from me for years and had therefore naturally become a huge part of my life. What if I decided to do something different or alter things slightly and my health got worse? What if it suddenly got better? What would people think? I wasn't sure that I could start from scratch and I didn't feel mentally prepared to face a lot of the responsibilities and lifestyle changes that come with being healthy and 'normal'. It was often easier just to stay cocooned in my room than meet family and friends and be prepared to face questions, such as, "Are you better now?" and "Have you been to the doctor?". I didn't have the heart or the energy to admit that I wasn't any better and that no-one had any answers for me, so staying away and keeping quiet seemed like the best option. It got to the point where I didn't want to speak with anyone about it for fear I'd drown in the disappointment and loss that was stirring and cultivating inside me. I didn't want to feel any sort of emotional connection with anyone for fear that I'd start crying and never be able to stop.

Even though a lot of my earlier anxieties and fears about my illness and the future had cleared since moving to Australia, I still needed to clear the stagnant energy I felt chained to, so I put a silent call out to the Universe for help.

A Welcome Turning Point

A few weeks later, I attended a Mind, Body, Spirit Festival in Sydney. I couldn't believe I was there, to be honest- this definitely wasn't the type of thing that was the norm in my tiny village back in the U.K, so I felt like a fraud and a little unsure of what to expect.

About an hour after arriving at the festival, I was just about to leave (I think I was freaked out by how much fun I was having and how natural it all felt), when I spotted an orange stand out of the corner of my eye. AcuEnergetics© were based literally along the road from where we lived and I had to laugh out loud at the coincidence of it all. Without really knowing what was happening, I had signed up for a 15-minute taster session, explaining that I'd been feeling run down and tired lately. For some reason, I didn't want to tell them about the CFS- keeping it quiet had become a habit and I didn't want to keep talking about it (new country, new life). I knew that these sessions were supposed to bring you back into balance energetically, to release blocks in your system and help your body to heal itself, but I had no idea what to expect and felt so nervous before trying it. I think I was secretly paranoid that someone I knew was going to come round the corner and see that what I was doing was a little too 'woo woo'.

Despite my anxiety, I lay down and closed my eyes for 15

minutes. When the energy healing session was over, I felt completely baffled. I felt different, but didn't know if it was in a good way or a bad way. Everything looked brighter. I stepped outside afterwards, and the light was so blinding that it almost knocked me over. It felt as though I was seeing things properly for the first time.

My legs and arms felt so light and free that I felt as though I was gliding along the road. I was smiling unabashedly at people who walked past and I was on a strange, but incredible, high.

I looked up the organisation when I returned home, and decided that I *had* to book in for further treatments. Even though this whole thing felt completely bizarre and almost ludicrous, it felt as though this was the answer I'd been looking for. I had no idea who to see, but just went with the first person with an available appointment.

Beautiful Ali Coleman is now one of my closest friends and mentors, and she has taught me so much about my condition, the possible root causes of it and how to get the most out of each energy healing session. Her grounded and gorgeous energy continue to inspire me, and she is such shining example of what living your truth really looks like.

One thing that became very clear from our sessions was that everything that I had intuited about my condition from Caroline Myss' book was completely right. I had been trying to hide away from the world, but was also harbouring a lot of anger for what had happened in the past. Anger is often said to be stored in the liver, which is why I had become jaundiced when I had glandular fever. This meant that I was still clinging on to a lot of stagnant, blocked energy, which was making it difficult for me to move on. Even the fall I had had which affected my hip showed how frightened I was to move on and change, and magnified the self-created beliefs about myself that I just couldn't (or wouldn't) move past. It seemed as though my mind was trying to hang on to the physical symptoms and pain I was exhibiting because I was frightened of what it would be like if I fully let the past go. It seemed as though it wasn't the present or the future I needed to worry about anymore, but the letting go of what was. I even moved to the other side of the world in an effort to rid myself of my past. I still struggle with letting things be as they are today, and I know this will be a constant learning curve in my life. Just because we maybe struggled with something once doesn't necessarily mean we can tick it off the list and be done with it. Destruction and creation are a constant part of life, a concept that I wasn't willing to accept or acknowledge in my younger years after my diagnosis.

I also suddenly realised what an expert I'd become at pushing away help. *Any* help that people would give me, I had to try and have the upper hand, because they didn't know what it was like for me. They didn't know how terrible I felt, and I didn't want to let anyone in in case they thought less of me (or I thought less of myself). My husband gave me so much good advice about prioritising myself when I relapsing, but whether through brain fog or just sheer bloody-mindedness, I couldn't take it on board until I was ready to.

Living the Lessons

During my sessions with Ali, more advice in the form of other self-help books just seemed to flow into my life, and there's still nothing I like better than really getting my teeth into a good book. I will also say here that even though I'm a huge fan of self-help books, I've realised recently that I've fallen into the trap of believing that there's something fundamentally wrong with me every time I read one of them.

Don't let self-help and spiritual books make you feel like any less of a person or that there is something wrong with you. Wherever you are right now is absolutely perfect, and to be honest, where else would you be?! These books are incredible tools which enable us to heal, gain perspective and find our place in the world, but you should mould the books to *you* rather than the other way around. With the vast choice and range of books out there, it's easy to fall down the rabbit hole- just when you're trying to fix one problem, it turns out that the problem you thought you had is actually indicative of *another* problem. Pretty soon it seems as though you're drowning in other problems, which is now causing a bigger problem than the one you came to self-help with!

Another thing we seem to forget, especially if we've been diagnosed with anything which completely flattens us and robs us of our energy, is that having energy for life is natural. We were born with it, so if our energy starts to come back to us, we need to believe and trust in it. It doesn't mean we should try to use it up as soon as we have it (a difficult lesson if you've been stuck in bed day after day), but we have to trust and believe that if it's here today, and if we're feeling and *witnessing* it today, that it'll still be here tomorrow. Even if you don't physically feel it in the way you expect to, you have acknowledged its presence in your body.

It took me until after I'd been completely healed to realise this, but our bodies are absolute miracles. We might not want to hear this when they're crying out in pain, but our bodies are incredible. Our heart has been beating since before we even arrived here. Our veins and arteries are thick with blood and goodness that is constantly serving us. Our organs are working in pure, unadulterated harmony without asking for anything in return. Our lungs help to filter out what we need and bring us even more precious life force.

Our bodies *are* healing us- they never cease to believe in us and are astoundingly intelligent. The least we can do is believe in them. I stopped acknowledging that my body and mind were one entity after my diagnosis. I believed that my body was broken, and the more my head convinced me of this, the worse my brain fog and physical symptoms got.

The lesson in all of this remains however that just because our bodies are broken doesn't mean that *we* are broken, as spirits and as humans. Your being here is no accident or happenstance. You still have all the dreams, triumphs and failures that everyone does, and being ill doesn't make you any less of a person or any less worthy of living an incredible life.

You are not broken.

Creation from Destruction

Although it seemed to be all wine and roses after I discovered energy healing, I knew that I had to create and believe in lasting change if I was to keep my good health going and it was up to me to implement what I had learned and walk through life as fearlessly and courageously as I was able.

It was very shortly after my final session with Ali that I started writing about what I'd experienced, from sleeping to supplements, from remorse to relapse. This is still what I feel many of us, CFS or no CFS, are doing on a daily basis-

summoning up strength that we didn't know we had in situations we never thought we'd find ourselves in. Sometimes we have to lose ourselves to find ourselves again, and the cycle continues, but meeting every fear or fearful emotion I encounter with curiosity and intrigue rather than sheer panic, as I'm naturally inclined to do, enables me to move through the world with a little more grace.

It helps me to take care of myself when I'm convinced that I haven't 'earned' it today, that I can't possibly sit down and relax when there's so much to do. Then I think back to my never-ending to-do list when I was teaching and know that we'll always have a to-do list, but that it's ok to prioritise your wellbeing and put yourself at the top of the list- unashamedly, with neon pink highlighter and sticky gold stars. I now feel as though I'm making up for lost time, and I'm consciously bringing this curiosity into how I treat and speak to myself in the same way I did with my illness. In speaking to and acknowledging my past illness, I was also able to speak to my true self. Again this is an ongoing practice, but one which continues to fascinate me on a daily basis.

The calm after the storm

I also decided to look into my diet a little more after my energy healing sessions. Having been vegetarian since my early teens, I presumed I had quite a healthy diet, but on closer inspection, there was hardly any good protein in it, which is essential for day-to-day energy and activity. Often putting things *into* your diet is a hell of a lot easier than taking things out. The trend for 'smoothie snapping' and a new diet being featured and/or criticised every week can make us wonder what in the world we're supposed to eat next.

My first experiment with nutrition was eliminating dairy, first and foremost because, to be frank, I always found the idea of drinking milk a little weird anyway. I've been dairy-free for about 5 years now, and I find that I don't feel as though I've got a clogged up throat or nose as often as I used to. However, I can't put my hand on my heart and say that I'm 100% gluten-free, although I try to avoid it and do notice a big difference in my stomach when I don't eat it. I haven't eliminated sugar completely either- the thought of giving up fruit makes me a little sad. The idea of going raw vegan is always incredibly appealing, but I've definitely got a body that craves warm foods (thanks Ayurveda!). The odd raw dessert is delicious, but my body can't handle too much raw goodness.

One thing that I also realised is that I used to just see food as fuel, not as something to be enjoyed. Food is meant to be a celebration, but for a number of years, probably because others were constantly making sure that I ate something (well, anything), I didn't see it that way. Another thing I came to realise is that although diet is naturally important, if we feel guilty because we lapsed or ate a big donut, then this negativity and abuse is almost worse for our bodies than the sugar or the fat in the donut. It's important to respect our bodies enough to nourish them as best we can, but also cultivating kindness and understanding in your mind and spirit are equally important. You can drink all the vegetable juice you want, but if you're still telling yourself you're useless, it's like throwing good money after bad.

I could spend pages upon pages advising you which diet might be right for you, but it's not rocket science (although there is a whole industry based around convincing people that it is).

My guideline, in the words of journalist, author and activist, Michael Pollan, is:

"Eat food. Not too much. Mostly plants."

Just do your best with where you are.

I also needed to re-examine my relationship to sleep. As blindingly obvious as it seems, I wasn't exempt from the basic human need for sleep. I wasn't a superhuman who lived on a diet of magic dust and could stay awake for weeks on end. Just because I'd spent what felt like years sleeping didn't mean I was suddenly able to stay awake for weeks at a time.

We all need sleep, so for goodness sakes, don't push it away or feel guilty for doing what humans instinctively need to do. Just because you have a fatigue-related illness doesn't mean you're not entitled to sleep like everyone else. About a year into my illness, I realised that I just wasn't that special- I needed sleep like everyone else and I would be an idiot to fight it.

CHAPTER 7
AN ONGOING EXPERIENCE

This isn't really a 'happy ever after story' where we close the book and skip off into the sunset. Even though I'm completely healed of CFS and I know that there are still many lessons to come from my time with it, I'm definitely in a much healthier place that I was this time 10 years ago.

Living in Sydney, with its incredible beaches and harbour, is helping me day-by-day to trust the value of play and having down-time, but it's sometimes more of a slog than it should be. This is going to sound terrible, but I'm not one who naturally goes for 'fun'. I think when you've spent 10 years of your life living in a small slice of hell, never knowing when you're going to see the end of it, there's a little part of you that doesn't want to have fun, 'just in case' you overexert yourself. I occasionally catch myself wondering if I'm going to have enough energy to make it through the day, but I know that this is just my ego wanting to hang on to that teeny, tiny part of me that still carries my 'sick person' story. I can drop these 'no energy' stories now quite easily and send them on their way by surrendering to the present moment. I'm definitely someone who worries about the future and what might happen, whereas my husband is someone who dwells on the past. We tend to balance each other out quite nicely in that way.

Unfortunately, one of the biggest lessons from my illness is also one of the saddest. I realised about two years ago that I was unconsciously pushing away joy and fun. I realised, with a very sorry heart, that I felt that CFS had turned me into a secretly 'serious' person. When I'm with friends or teaching, I'm fun, energetic and spirited, but I often tend to avoid spontaneous activities, again, because I think we plan and pre-empt everything so meticulously when we're ill. We need to plan for relapse and disappointment, we need to avoid certain situations and surprises just in case, and in my case the most draining situations, which also require a certain degree of spontaneity, are social situations.

Don't get me wrong, I'm not a hermit living in a cave, but I learned the hard way, through constant relapses, that pushing myself to my limits just wasn't worth it. I had to define what my limits were and they definitely don't look like other peoples'. I used to see this as 'wimping out' and I was terrified that others would think I wasn't fun enough, or that I couldn't let my hair down because I don't drink. My friends don't think any less of me if I duck away at 9pm instead of 1am- it doesn't make a blind bit of difference to their evening. Eventually though, I realised that my boundaries are just that- *my* boundaries. It is not for me to compare myself to anyone else, or question their opinion of me. In the incredible words of Dr. Wayne Dyer, "What other people think of me is none of my business." You have so much going on in your own body just trying to heal that you can't waste energy on what other people think of you.

Ultimately, living with a debilitating illness for 10 years affects you even if you don't consciously realise it- there's no way that you'll be exactly the same person as when you started out. Clinging onto our past reality can cause even more anxiety and puts stress on our bodies, so accepting our state becomes truly liberating and enhances our well-being. Our bodies are constantly changing, so it's wise to accept that our thoughts and lives are too. Nothing can stay completely static for too long.

I am not perfect. I am definitely not flawless blogger with a textbook Instagram profile (and therefore, a perfect life). We often think that when we're fully recovered, everything in our life will magically snap into place, but my battle scars are still with me, frequently tripping me up and trying to keep me small. Every time they do, I say 'thank you', as they guide me to become aware of those not-so-shiny parts. One of the biggest takeaways from my illness is that being uncomfortable and feeling strong enough to meet your 'darkness' head on takes a hell of a lot of guts. I think that's why I avoided it for so long. It's even worse when friends and relatives have no idea what you're going through, but then again, how can we really expect them to truly understand everything *exactly* as we're seeing and experiencing it? You're the lone warrior moving through territory that could either make or break you, and you have no idea what you're going to find on the other side of it.

This is when we discover we need to drop our idea of what 'perfect healing' looks like. It's not sparkling and polished- it's messy, chaotic and often frantic with a knotty head of hair and dirt beneath its fingernails. We are not the girl sitting in an idyllic, beautiful field of perfect green grass on a perfect summer's day meditating for hours on end, wearing the gorgeous dress and allowing all that is good to come to us. We struggle, push, pull and meddle in the hope that we know better than anything else that is out there. We project our own idealised version of healing on to our own life and suddenly become very disappointed when we realise that what we thought it should look like isn't actually what we're presented with. More disturbingly, what we thought *we* would look and feel like isn't what we imagined it to be at the 'end'.

The truth is, there is no 'end'. We are all beautifully and agonisingly human, with flaws and foibles, and after healing, in whatever form that takes for you, there will *still* be pitfalls, and that contrast of the good and the not so good. We keep moving the goalposts, but there will always be an aim, an ideal, a utopia. Our work is never truly finished, so maybe healing is never truly finished either. My illness was long, agonising and bumpy, and took around 10 years to play out, but yours will not look exactly like mine. To be honest, I wouldn't want it to. Whatever you're going through now is meant for you, and you only. I've read about people who healed themselves in a matter of months and people who've been ill for 50 years- everything is as it is. Comparing ourselves to others, especially in a wellness industry in which people are touting the latest instant miracle cure or programme, is becoming more common and we want what everyone else has got. Eventually, we come to forget what it really is that's true and authentic for us.

At the beginning of our illness, once we're well enough, we spend a lot of our time looking outside of ourselves for the answers, because we trust that someone has been there before, they've had our experiences and therefore, there must be a cure or obvious solution. We want to find out about supplements, treatments, articles and books that could help us on the way. This is all well and good, but sooner or later, we discover that we have our own individual energetic pattern, and we have to know that looking outside of ourselves might not always bring us the answers that we want. I found out very early on in my illness that I had to stop reading medical articles and journals related to CFS, as not only did the medical language make my brain fog worse, but in looking for answers, I seemed to convince myself that there really was no answer and therefore, I was destined to stay sick. Of course, medical journals, research, doctors and diet can help, but in the end, even if they give us the magic pill, it's all down to us. How we move through the world, how we handle our energy, how we interact with others- it's all on us and it's our divine responsibility to do with it what we are guided to do.

Many people email me looking for the silver bullet, the 'one thing' I did to help me heal. I've had clients who become a little angry when I can't give them the answer they're looking for, and I completely understand why. We want something to take the pain away, so we can feel like a real person again as quickly and as effortlessly as possible, without other people seeing us struggle and having to, embarrassingly, psyche ourselves up for the baby steps. We want to have just *one day* of feeling like we fit in and that we can blend in with the routines of the rest of humanity, hence the reason we fling ourselves out the door at the mere *hint* of an increase in energy. We want connection and sometimes we find that serenity and togetherness in the mundane, the totally ordinary.

One of the traps I got myself into however was feeling like this was never enough for me. Walking 200 metres to the supermarket wasn't enough for one day when everyone else could go to work, put in a full day in stressful environments, do some grocery shopping and still have the energy for a social life. Therefore, if my actions weren't enough, *I* wasn't enough either. Even though we barely know someone we see on the street or on social media, we instinctively compare ourselves to them. We want to know what's possible and 'normal', but forget that we're often projecting our version of perfection onto the lives of total strangers. We don't shout about the bits we don't want others to see.

In many ways, for a number of years, I was ashamed that I was able to come home at a reasonable time and avoid the rush hour because of my job. I was convinced that if it was all too easy that I'd dropped the ball somewhere and it wasn't ok. It meant that I was less of a person and had to make up for it in other areas of my life. I was letting my ego push in and tell me that I was only worthy and deserving of relaxing if my calendar was chock full to the max, I had a to-do list that was longer than my arm, I had 'this much' in my bank account and I was pushing myself to the very edges of what my body was energetically capable of. This is why I was so fascinated with my mentor who went swimming every evening after school. How could she be so self-indulgent in the face of such a stressful job? I've learned the hard way that there are no prizes for burnout and self-loathing, and what might work for one person might fall flat on its face with you.

Stress, late nights and frenzy are not sexy. Respect yourself enough to acknowledge that life *can* be easy if you allow it to be. It is what it is.

It all hangs on the existence of opposites- if there is perfection, there must also be imperfection. The cycle of the Earth rotates around darkness and light, and it is therefore somewhat naive and foolhardy to think that our healing journey will be plain-sailing and sparkly. We need *both* for the full human experience, and that's why, even though I've done a lot of inner work to get me to where I am today, I still carry the scars from my illness. They remind me of the importance of truth in all things and that I am forever a student of life and the Universe.

The Light at the End of the Tunnel

When did I realise I was completely better?

When I stopped putting my illness before all my wants and desires. I realised that I hadn't thought about CFS for months. I was able to go to yoga and go hiking without worrying about whether or not I had the energy to get through it. I was able to go with how I was feeling in the moment, rather than how I *thought* I was going to feel the day after if I did x, y, z today.

I always dreamed of waking up one morning and experiencing some kind of glorious, angelic vision telling me that my body was totally healed. I fantasised about how my first day as a 'healthy person' would look and what I would do with my newfound energy. This didn't happen to me, but the alternative was so much more satisfying and rewarding. I remember the day I suddenly realised that I hadn't experienced any pain or fatigue in months, and it was one of the strangest feelings I've ever encountered. I shut myself in the bathroom, fell on the floor and cried. Whether it was in relief, sadness or sheer joy, it didn't matter. I suddenly tuned into my body and just knew that I'd made peace with it, with everything. I had stepped out of my own way enough to trust my body and it had replied in kind through a supreme sense of wellbeing.

I haven't had a cold or the flu in 5 years, and visits to the doctor are few and far between. Sometimes I can't believe that the person popping every vitamin under the sun and spending an unfathomable amount of time in doctor's waiting rooms was me. But it was, and I hope that by sharing my story, you'll be able to realise that healing is very possible for you too.

CHAPTER 8
CLOSING

If there's anything that you can take from my lessons and where I went wrong then I'm grateful to be of service. Even though I've been in great health for over 5 years now, I'm still connecting the dots. I'm still piecing together that big chunk of my twenties that went missing and trying not to get too caught up in what could've been. I'm here, perfectly imperfect, and taking it day-by-day like everyone else.

I still find myself saying, 'I'm tired', when what I actually want to say is 'no' or 'I can't be bothered', a phrase there's no crime in saying. I still find myself saying, 'I don't know' or 'I'm not sure' when I've really just lost connection to my own power and sense of self.

I still sing in the shower. In a world of triathlons, I still prefer walking to any other form of exercise. I'm still obsessed with all things French. I'm still terrible at cooking, but not so bad at baking. I still don't like having my photo taken, and I still can't resist doing handstands on deserted beaches.

All I want to say is this:

You will find your own way out of this. There is life after this illness.

I would've loved a silver bullet, or for someone to tell me exactly how to heal, but I'd have been robbed of an incredible learning curve. Unfortunately, nobody gives us the blueprints to navigate every step of life, and healing is no different.

When you look back, all your experiences during your illness will be quite memorable, and maybe not for the reasons you thought they would be, but you cannot shut yourself off.

Leave yourself open and always try to look for the good in whatever crappy situation you might find yourself in. This is when the books start to fall off the shelves, when your intuition is too loud to be ignored and when you stop comparing where you are to where you believe other people are.

Give yourself a little credit, my lovely. I see you.

You're still in the game.

♥

"And the day came when the risk to remain tight in a bud was more painful than the risk it took to blossom."

- Anaïs Nin

CHAPTER 9
RESOURCES

Books

- 'You Can Heal Your Life' - Louise Hay
- 'Anatomy of the Spirit' - Caroline Myss
- 'Daring Greatly' - Brené Brown
- 'How To Stop Worrying and Start Living' - Dale Carnegie
- 'In Defense of Food: An Eater's Manifesto' - Michael Pollan

Websites

- Ali Coleman: http://www.alicoleman.com.au/
- AcuEnergetics©: http://www.acuenergetics.com

ABOUT THE AUTHOR

Katie Manning is a writer, teacher, mentor and speaker and the creator of the blog, 'Conquering Fear Spiritually'. The blog documents the steps she took to completely heal herself of a 10-year illness with M.E./CFS (Chronic Fatigue Syndrome). After being free of the illness for over five years, Katie inspires others to take control of their own healing journey and live healthy, peaceful lives, free from chronic illness.

Katie helps her clients and readers to remember who they really are without CFS or chronic illness. She endeavours to live by her own teachings, and loves to investigate how fear plays a part in our lives physically, emotionally and spiritually.

www.conqueringfearspiritually.com

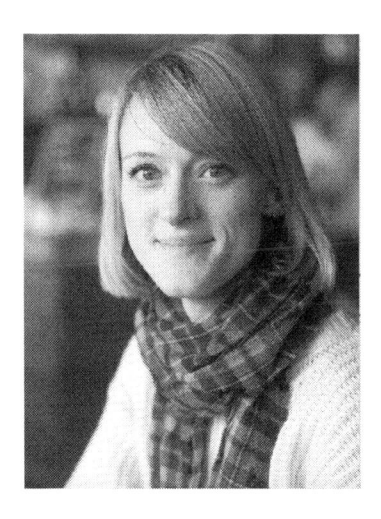

Printed in Great Britain
by Amazon